1

Shen Long Publishing
www.shenlongpub.com

To My First Taiji Teacher

Thank you for your teaching
and your friendship.

Acknowledgments

Many thanks to my friends who
shared this Qi Gong
system with me.

Table of Contents

Introduction

Qi 氣

Qi is not something mysterious. It is all around us and animates everything including ourselves even if we are not aware of it. The most common translation for Qi (氣) is Energy and it is pronounced "chee."

According to Traditional Chinese Medical Theory, Qi has different functions in the body and can be classified as different types of Qi depending on what function it is carrying out. Each organ has its own Qi because each organ has a certain function. The simplest and least esoteric way to look at and define Qi would be to say that Qi is the "functional" aspect of anything.

While there are many different types of Qi in the body, we take in or receive energy from only two main sources. One is finite and we inherit this from our parents and the universe at the time of our conception and the other we can constantly replenish through lifestyle, diet, and exercise. These two types of energy are classified as Pre-Heaven and Post-Heaven respectively.

Chinese theory states that we receive Energy from our parents when we are conceived. Because this Energy is given to us before we are born it is called Pre-Heaven Qi or Energy. In a western sense this type of Energy or Qi can be seen as our genetic makeup. This Energy is finite and can only be worn away or depleted with time.

After we are born we get our nourishment from the food we eat and the air we breathe. Our body processes the food and air to get all the nutrients and substances we need to keep our body healthy. This is called Post-Heaven Qi or Energy because this is how we nourish ourselves after we are born. Through Qi Gong exercise we can enhance the way the body takes in energy from the environment (breathing and digestion) and the way energy is utilized.

Each organ in the body has a different function and the Qi of the organ is said to carry out this function.
Our organs are not independent things but instead they interact and depend on each other. When they are functioning properly they are in harmony. If the function of one organ is impaired it can effect the functional aspect of other organs.

Additionally each organ has its own energy pathway. These pathways are called meridians. The energy of the organ runs through these pathways and these pathways also connect with other meridians. This is another way that the organs are interrelated and connected. When an Acupuncturist places a needle into a meridian he or she is accessing the energy of that pathway and by doing so also the energy of the related organ. Because these pathways travel over every part of the body, exercise can also help to stimulate these pathways. Certain exercises and movements can also be used to stimulate specific meridians and organs.

In addition to the organs and meridians our body also has three centers or collection points. These are called Dan Tien, which translates as field of elixir. Inside our body these fields are a place for cultivation. As the name suggests the cultivation process is similar to the way crops are cultivated in a field, with much care for making sure the environment is right for cultivation but not much meddling in the actual process of transformation. If you grow a plant you can make sure the soil is fertile and that the seedling gets air, water, and sun. But the plant grows on its own. You can not really help it along, you can only observe the changes and transformations that take place and adjust the conditions accordingly. For personal practice this would relate to a healthy lifestyle, good nutrition, and consistent practice. Over time the transformations in the body will take place naturally.

These three centers house what are called the Three Treasures: Jing, Qi, and Shen.

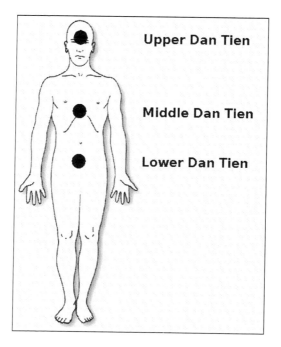

The Lower Dan Tien is located about 2-3 inches below the umbilicus and at the center of the body. This center is associated with Jing. Jing is the most coarse substance of the three and relates to the physical body. Jing is often translated into English as sperm and is the origin of life.

The Middle Dan Tien is located in the middle of the chest at about the level of the solar plexus. This center is associated with Qi or Energy. This center also relates to the mind.

The Upper Dan Tien is located in the head and is related to Shen. Shen is thought of as spirit or consciousness.

The Three Treasures (Jing, Qi, and Shen) are all related and can support and transform into each other. They are actually the same substance at different levels of refinement.

Shen is more refined/rarefied Qi.
Qi is more refined/rarefied Jing.

Once Jing becomes abundant it will transform into Qi.
Once Qi becomes abundant it will transform into Shen.

The three treasures relate to practice in that they emphasize the physical training first. The body is the same as a container that must be filled from the bottom up. This means that in order to practice safely and avoid problems always start by having a strong physical foundation through training. Once this strong foundation is achieved the mind and spirit will be supported and healthy. With a strong foundation we can achieve higher goals in cultivation. If the foundation of physical work is neglected the energy in the body can become ungrounded. The Five Animal Frolics are a very good practice for building a strong foundation.

Qi Gong 氣功

Qi (氣) means Energy and Gong (功) means Work..Literally Qi Gong means exercises that work with the body's Energy or Qi. Qi Gong training has a very long history going back thousands of years. Over this long period of time many refinements have been made and many different exercises have been developed. Even though there are many different types of Qi Gong exercise most have a common goal. This goal is to harmonize the posture, breath, and mind. When this harmony is achieved it allows well-being and health to manifest. It is the disharmony of our internal body including the stagnation of Qi that creates disease and pain (both physical and emotional).

Qi Gong is a way for us to keep our body in harmony and take control of our health and well-being. Qi Gong can be practiced almost anywhere. It does not require lots of space or any fancy machines or equipment. The gentle, non-strenuous, circular movements work to twist our body and joints, not only stimulating our physical body of tendons, muscle, and organs but also our energetic pathways or meridians. This stimulation helps to maintain the free flow of Qi and Blood and break up any stagnation that might exist.

This free flow of Qi and Blood helps to ensure that the body gets the nourishment that it needs to functional at its optimal level as well as recuperate. Not only is the functioning enhanced but the body's capacity to store and use Qi will also expand.

The Five Animal Frolics 五禽戲

The Five Animal Frolics were created by Hua Tuo (circa 200AD). Hua Tuo was a very famous physician and had mastered many facets of medicine including surgery. Hua Tuo understood that treating disease was only a small part of medicine and well-being. Instead, prevention is the key. By studying nature he was able to devise five sets of exercises that mimic the movements of the animals. These exercises keep the Qi and blood moving freely, strengthen the body, increase range of motion, and reduce stress and tension held in the body.

Because these exercises have such a long history there exist many variations of these exercises. Some versions have single exercises for each animal or many exercises for each animal, some versions mimic the movements and characteristics of each animal, and some versions do not seem to relate to the animals at all except in name.

The following is excerpted from "Kung Fu, or Taoist Medical Gymnastics" by John Dudgeon. It was published in Tientsin by the Tientsin Press in 1895.[1] It is included to serves as an example of an ancient set of Five Animal Frolics that is composed of a single exercise for each animal. Also included is a brief introduction.

> *These figures for the cure of disease by perspiration were designed by the celebrated surgeon Hwa-to, of the Han dynasty (2nd century A.D.), who is not only the Esculapius of China but was well versed in all the secrets of Taoism. He was wondrously skilled in acupuncture, and*

---

1 This work falls within public domain in the US as it was published before 1923. Text and images taken from www.sacred-texts.com.

some of his surgical operations are of a very marvelous description. He was. the first to use anesthetics in scraping the poison from the arm of Kwan-ti, the god of war and patron of the present dynasty. If one's body is not in health and peace, the performance of these five figures will produce perspiration and cure the disease and discomfort.

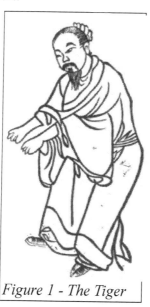

Figure 1 - The Tiger

Figure 1.—The Tiger. Close the breath, bend the head, close the fists tightly, and assume the severe form of a tiger. The two hands are slowly to lift a supposed weight of 1000 catties; the breath is to be retained till the body is upright, then swallowed and carried down into the abdomen. This is to cause the "divine air" (animal spirits, energy) to proceed from above downwards and produce in the abdomen a sound like thunder; to be done some 7 times. By this sort of movement, the air and pulses of the body will be harmonized, and the hundred (all) diseases prevented from being produced.

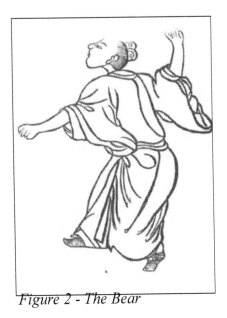

Figure 2 - The Bear

Figure 2.—The Bear. Assume the form of a bear, incline the body slightly to the side, swing it to the right and left, place one foot in front and one behind, and stand fast. Use the air till the ribs on the two sides and the joints all resound. Also, move the strength of the loins to remove the swelling (?) some 3 to 5 times. This will relax and tranquilize the tendons and bones. This also is the method for nourishing the blood.

18

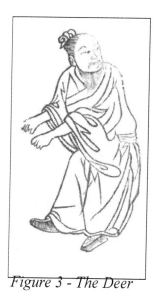

Figure 3 - The Deer

Figure 3.—The Deer. Shut the breath, bend the head, close the fists tightly, turn the head like a deer viewing its tail; the body even, contract the shoulders, stand on tip-toe, stamp on the heel, and including the "heavenly pillar" (the neck) the entire body will move; do it some 3 times, or each day once will also do. To do it once, on getting out of bed in the morning, is the best of all.

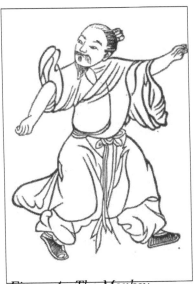
Figure 4 - The Monkey

Figure 4.—The Monkey. Stop the breath, assume
the form of a monkey climbing a tree, one hand
as it were holding some fruit, one foot raised; on
the heel of one foot turn the body, and cause the
"divine air" to revolve, carrying it into the
abdomen till you feel perspiration is .exuding,
and then it is finished.

20

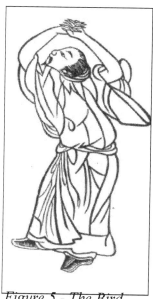

Figure 5 - The Bird

Figure 5.—The Bird. Close the breath, assume the form of a bird flying, raise the head, inspire the air of the coccyx, and cause it to ascend to the hollow of the vertex (head); let the two hands assume in front [the   attitude of] reverence [or worship], raise the head (so as to have the face upwards), and go out to meet the spirit and break the vertex (i.e., open the brain, as it were, to receive it).

In contrast the the above quoted text, the version of the Five Animal Frolics that I learned and present in this book has multiple exercises for each animal and mimics some of the characteristics of the animals themselves.

The two sets presented in this book are suitable for most people to practice and when practiced together they complement each other and form a rather complete practice.

I do not know the history of the Five Animal Frolics that I learned and present partially in this book. They were taught to me by some good friends who learned them from their teacher. I got to met their teacher briefly before he moved away but the history of the set past that is unknown to me. I chose to continue to practice these sets and to share them because I feel that they are very good sets with many benefits.

My friends learned the Five Animal Frolics as part of their Taiji training. I agree that these sets can be a great compliment to Taiji practice. The two sets presented in this book can make a great foundation for further Taiji practice. As stated before they are the sets most suitable for the majority of people to practice. The remaining sets (Deer, Monkey, and Tiger) are also good but might not be for everyone because some of the exercises require some strength and flexibility to preform.

Five Elements 五行

This is a brief introduction to the Chinese theory of the Five Elements or Wu Xing. The Five Elements are Wood, Fire, Earth, Metal, and Water. The Five Elements are a Chinese concept that can be used to describe almost everything and also the relationship between things.

The Five Elements have the following correspondences:

	Metal	Water	Wood	Fire	Earth
Color	White	Dark Blue	Green	Red	Yellow
Direction	West	North	East	South	Center
Yin Organ	Lungs	Kidney	Liver	Heart	Spleen
Yang Organ	Large Intestine	Urinary Bladder	Gall-bladder	Small Intestine	Stomach
Season	Autumn	Winter	Spring	Summer	Transition between Seasons
Emotion	Grief	Fear	Anger	Joy	Worry
Tastes	Pungent	Salty	Sour	Bitter	Sweet
Sense Organ	Nose	Ears	Eyes	Tongue	Mouth
Tissues	Skin	Bones	Sinews	Vessels	Muscles

It must be remembered that the Five Elements do not exist by themselves but instead form a whole and as such the relationship between the elements are very important. The two main relationships between the Five Elements are expressed through the generating cycle and the controlling cycle.

In the Generating Sequence each Element generates another Element. This relationship is sometimes referred to as the Mother and Son Relationship. Metal generates Water. Water generates Wood. Wood generates Fire. Fire generates Earth. Earth generates Metal. In this relationship the Element that generates the other is referred to as the Mother Element and it nourishes the Son Element which is being generated. In this relationship the mother gives energy to the son but the son also draws energy from the mother. The generating sequence is represented in the following illustration:

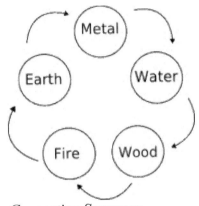

Generating Sequence

In the Controlling Sequence one Element controls another Element. Metal controls Wood. Wood controls Earth. Earth controls Water. Water controls Fire. Fire controls Metal. The controlling sequence is represented in the following illustration:

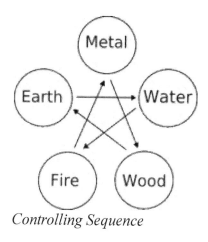

Controlling Sequence

It is interesting to note that because there are five elements there can never be a one to one correlation between them. If we look at the illustration of the Controlling Sequence we will see that each Element controls another and that the Element that is being controlled also generates the Element that controls the original Element. For example Water controls Fire and Fire generates Earth. Earth controls Water. This is just an example of how the relationship between the Elements can be explored. If we look at the Five Element Correlation Chart we can see that these relationships can be used to describe the natural world or the workings of the internal body.

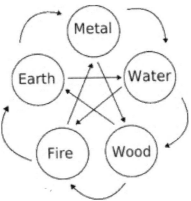

Five Element Interactions

Only a brief introduction of Five Element Theory is related in this text. To delve into the intricacies of this symbolic model and the implications and knowledge that can be gained by studying it would take a complete text unto itself. Also a complete understanding of this model is not necessary for the practice of the Five Animal Frolics Qi Gong.

The Five Animal Frolics and the Five Elements

Each of the five sets of exercises that compose the five animal frolics relates to one of the Five Elements. Although the Five Elements are a Chinese concept that can be used to describe almost everything and also the relationship between things, for this Qi Gong practice the Five Elements are used to represent which organ system the exercises are focusing one.

There are two things to note:

First:
Although each set of exercises focuses on a specific organ system, the organ systems are related and their proper functioning depends upon each other. Each organ can not be thought of as independent from the rest. Also too much focus on only one organ system can be harmful because it can unbalance the system.

The two sets taught in this book are the most balanced of the five sets in that they benefit more of the whole body. These two sets also balance each other out very nicely. The two sets presented in this book if practiced correctly can form a safe and very complete Qi Gong practice.

Second:
To benefit from these exercises you do not have to understand anything about Chinese Medical Theory or Five Element Theory. The benefit comes from the practice of the exercises and not theorizing about them.

The order in which the exercises are learned and what they correspond to:

Exercise	Element	Direction	Color	Season
Crane	Fire	South	Red	Summer
Bear	Water	North	Blue	Winter
Deer	Earth	Center	Yellow	Transition Between Seasons
Monkey	Wood	East	Green	Spring
Tiger	Metal	West	White	Fall

The Crane exercises strengthen the Heart organ system and benefits the circulation and lungs.

The Bear exercises strengthen the Kidney and Urogenital systems and benefits all the internal organs and the digestion.

The Deer exercises strengthen the Spleen organ system, help to relax the muscles, and make the body nimble.

The Monkey exercises strengthen the Liver organ system and benefits the tendons and ligaments.

The Tiger exercises strengthen the Lung organ system and help to develop a strong body.

How to Practice

As stated earlier, the Crane and the Bear exercises balance each other and can form a complete practice. When learning these sets it is normal to feel an affinity to one set over the other, but both sets should be practiced to maintain balance.

Both sets can be done in the same daily training period. Or, one can be done in the morning and the other at night. Or, they can be alternated on each training session. Or, they can be practiced according to the seasons. That is: more of the Crane set in the spring and summer and more of the Bear set in the fall and winter.

The most important thing though is to enjoy the practice.

When learning these sets, start with the Crane exercises. Once you can go through the Crane exercises without the aid of the book, practice them for a couple weeks. Then go back to the book and make sure you are performing each exercise correctly.

Then go on to learn the Bear exercises the same way.

To make sure you are performing the exercises correctly, please periodically check the book, even if you are performing both sets regularly.

Do:
Practice in a quite, natural, and clean setting
Wear loose and comfortable clothing
Allow yourself enough time so that you can practice
without watching the clock
Practice the complete set of exercises unless it is
indicated that it is OK to practice an exercise
individually

Don't:
Eat right before or after you practice
Practice on a full or empty stomach
Practice when upset or angry
Practice while under the influence of drugs/alcohol
Use the bathroom right after you practice
Expose yourself to a draft either while practicing or
right after practicing
Do strenuous activity when pregnant or menstruating

Please wait at least 45 minutes after you finish practicing
to either eat or to bathe.

Do not practice to the point of exhaustion. When you
finish these exercises you should feel invigorated and
refreshed, not tired and needing a break. The idea is to
improve your health and strength over time. When you
are practicing do only as much as is comfortable.

Do not do more than the recommended number of
repetitions. More is not always better.

For all of the exercises the breathing is in and out through
the nose. The breathing should be natural and never
strained or held. The breathing is directed to the lower
abdomen. For details please refer to the Breathing Crane
exercise, page 47. This way of breathing will become
natural with practice.

The tongue should be curled up so the tip is touching the upper palette. This makes a connection between two of the most important energy channels or meridians in the body (the Ren and the Du channels). These channels run up the back and down the front of the body at the midline.

With the tongue at the roof of the mouth, the body's energy can circulate naturally through these two channels. This circulation will happen all by itself even if you do not feel anything.

Remember to keep the body relaxed while performing these exercises. The shoulders and the elbows must always be relaxed. This relaxed state must be maintained even when the hands are brought higher than the shoulders. Make sure the shoulders are not hunched upwards and make sure the elbows are always pointing down. If too much tension is held in the shoulders while practicing it will be difficult to sink the breath into the lower abdomen.

When the breath is not directed to the lower abdomen it is very hard for the body to relax.

Remember that these sets are considered Qi Gong but at no time during the practice are we directing the Internal Energy or Qi. The practice of directing Qi with the mind can cause problems. That is why nowhere in any of the instructions does it say anything about this.

When you practice you might experience Qi moving inside your body. Don't be alarmed but at the same time do not try to duplicate or look for the same experience in future practice sessions. Merely observe the sensations and let go of them. Continual practice of any movement art should put you more deeply in touch with your body over time.

Concentrating or trying to duplicate a certain experience can hinder progress and further development.

Have fun when you practice. Remember that these sets are part of the Five Animal Frolics and not the Five Animals at Work. You should have the same carefree feeling that an animal has when it is playing. But, at the same time remember to perform all the exercises correctly.

Crane Frolics
Qi Gong

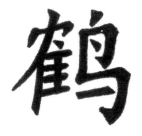

Introduction

The Crane Frolics Qi Gong Exercises consist of gentle, flowing movements that imitate a Crane moving its wings.

The Crane exercises belong to the Fire element and strengthen the Heart, Lungs, and circulation.

These exercises should be preformed in a relaxed manner. Coordinate the breathing with the movements. Make sure that you never become out of breath, force the breath, or hold the breath while practicing.

Please review and become familiar with the basic hand positions and the Crane Stance before beginning to learn these exercises.

Hand Positions

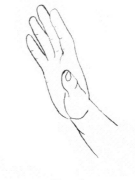

Fig-1

Palm

The fingers are naturally extended and the center of the palm should be slightly hollow. (Fig-1)

The hand should not be too straight or stiff or too curved or bent.

Extending the fingers in this way lets the Qi and the blood flow to the extremities of the body.

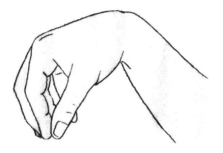

Fig-2

Crane's Beak

Bring the tips of you fingers and thumb together. (Fig-2)

Notice how the hand in this position looks like the head of a Crane.

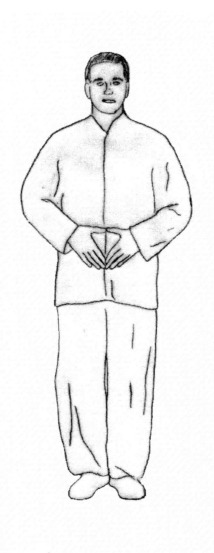

40

Crane Stance

Stand with the body straight and the heels touching. The toes should be pointed out so that the feet form an angle between 60-90 degrees.

Bend the knees slightly and relax the pelvis so that it naturally drops forward slightly, straightening the lower back. Note: The knees should always be in line with the toes throughout these exercises. (Fig-3)

Curl the tongue upwards so that the tip touches the upper palette.

Place your hands on your stomach. The thumbs and the index fingers are touching so that the hands form a triangle with the thumbs at the bellybutton and the fingers pointing down.

Men can keep their fingers together. (Fig-4)

Women can separate their pinky from the other fingers so that it falls over the ovaries. (Fig-5)

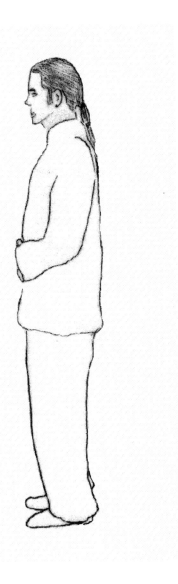

As you stand in this position try to feel that your spine is elongated by both stretching up and down. This stretching feeling is very subtle and should not be forced.

By relaxing your hips and letting your pelvis drop down and naturally forward you are lengthening the lower part of your spine. When the pelvis drops naturally forward the hips should be tucked slightly as if you were about to sit. Again there should be no tension in the hips.

To stretch the upper parts of the spine try to imagine that you are suspended from above. Let the entire body relax and "hang" as if by a string. Make sure that there is no tension in the neck. The proper position for the neck is with the chin pushed back and slightly down as if you are trying to touch the back of the neck to your shirt collar.

Make sure the knees are slightly bent and not straight. When the knees are slightly bent it is easier to open and relax the hip joints.

Do not bend the knees too much. The knees should not extend past the toes.

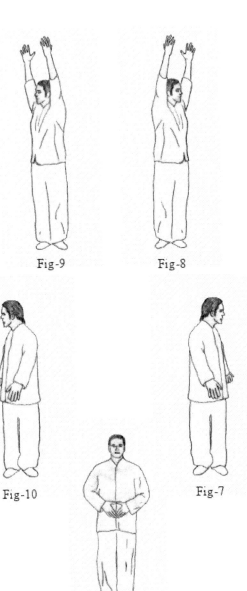

Fig-9

Fig-8

Fig-10

Fig-7

Fig-6

44

1. Windmill Crane

Start in the Crane Stance. (Fig-6)
Turn the upper body to the left. Inhale as you raise the hands up to over the head. (Fig-7) Your upper body should now be facing to the left side. The right hand moves up towards the front and the left hand up towards the back. As the hands move upward the palms face the ground. As the hands come over the head the fingertips point up and the palms turn to face each other. (Fig-8)

With the hands over the head turn the upper body to the right. (Fig-9) Exhale and lower the hands. The upper body should be facing to the right side and the right hand should move down towards the back and the left hand should move down towards the front. As the hands move down the palms face towards the ground. (Fig-10) Turn the upper body back to the left side and repeat the movement a total of 3 to 5 times.

After completing the last repetition return to the Crane Stance. (Fig-6) Then repeat the sequence on the other side by turning to the right and raising the arms as you inhale. The movements are the same but the direction is reversed. Repeat on this side 3-5 times. Then return to the Crane Stance (Fig-6)

As you move the hands imagine and feel the resistance of the air as if your arms were the wings of a Crane. As you inhale you can raise the body by straightening the legs slightly. As you exhale you can lower the body by bending the knees slightly. The body movement, arm movement, and breath should all be coordinated.

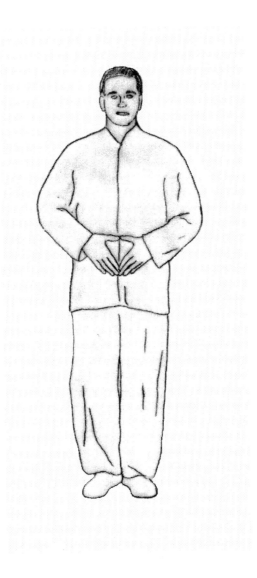

2. Breathing Crane

This form looks simple but has many benefits.

Stand in the Crane Stance and concentrate on your breathing. (Fig-11)

As you inhale imagine that the air comes all the way down to the lower stomach and starts to fill the body from the bottom up. The abdomen will naturally expand as you inhale. Try not to expand or move the chest as you inhale but instead concentrate on the abdomen "filling" with air.

As you exhale the abdomen will relax to its original position. The breathing must not be forced or strained in any way. Gradually over time the breath will get longer and deeper but do not force it. The breathing should also be so quiet that you can not even hear it yourself.

When the hands are at the lower abdomen it is easier to feel if you are doing this exercise correctly. After you are comfortable with this exercise, this breathing can be practiced anywhere and at anytime. When practicing this exercise separately from the set the hands do not need to be placed on the lower abdomen. This breathing can also be practiced while sitting or lying.

Breathing in this manner ensures that more of the air in the lungs is exchanged with each breath. As the abdomen expands on the inhale what is really happening is the diaphragm is relaxing downward to let the lungs expand fully. Over time the length of each breath should be increased naturally. Practicing this exercise will strengthen the lungs and permit optimum gaseous exchange, improve circulation, and stimulate the digestive organs.

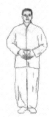

Fig-12

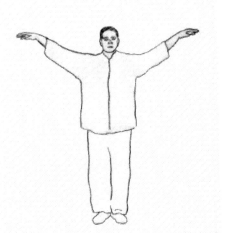

Fig-13

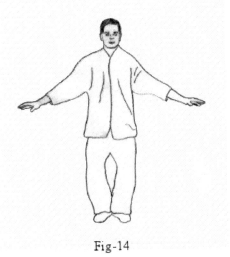

Fig-14

48

3. Soaring Crane

A. Soaring Crane I

Start in the Crane Stance. (Fig-12)

Inhale and raise the arms up the sides, palm facing down until the hands are about level with the head. (Fig-13)

Exhale and lower the arms until they are about level with the hips. (Fig-14)

To repeat this exercise, inhale and raise the arms up the sides palm down until they are about level with the top of the head. (Fig-13)

Repeat this movement 3-5 times. On the last exhale you will then move on to the next exercise.

As you inhale and raise the arms you can also raise the body by straightening the legs slightly. As you exhale and lower the arms you can lower the body by bending the knees slightly.

Feel the resistance of the air on your arms as if your arms were the wings of a crane.

Match the speed of the movement to the breath.

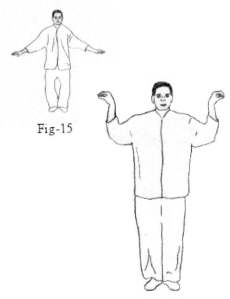

Fig-15

Fig-16

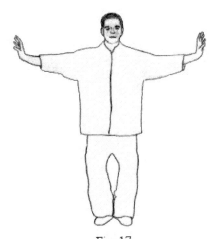

Fig-17

B. Soaring Crane II

Continue from the last exercise. (Fig-15)

Inhale and bring your fingertips and your thumb together to form a crane's beak as you pull your hands in towards your head. Your fingertips and elbows should be pointing to the sides. (Fig-16)

Exhale and push you palms out to the side at about shoulder level. (Fig-17)

Repeat this movement 3 to 5 times. On the last exhale you will move on to the next exercise.

As you inhale you can slightly raise the body by straightening the legs and as you exhale you can bend the knees slightly to lower the body.

Again match the speed of the movement to the breathing. Feel the resistance of the air as you move your arms and body.

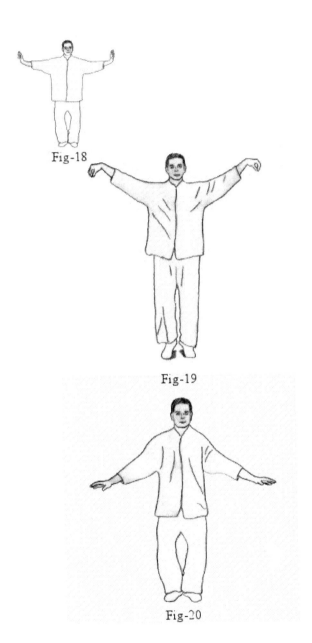

Fig-18

Fig-19

Fig-20

52

C. Soaring Crane III

Continue from the last exercise. (Fig-18)

Inhale and form a Crane's Beak with your fingers and raise your arms so that your hands are at the level of the head. As you raise your arms lift your heels off the ground. The fingertips should be pointing to the floor. (Fig-19)

Exhale lower your heels back to the ground and open your hands and lower them to about hip level as you bend your knees slightly. (Fig-20)

Repeat this movement 3 to 5 times. On the last one as you exhale you will go directly into the next exercise.

The body movement, arm movement, and breath should all be coordinated. Again match the speed of the movement to the breathing. Feel the resistance of the air as you move your arms and body.

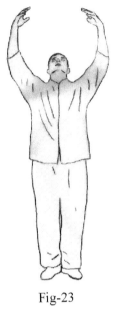

Fig-23

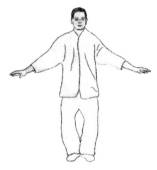

Fig-21

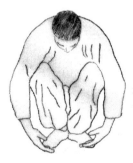

Fig-22

54

4. Squatting Crane

A. Squatting Crane I (Crane Washing Itself)

Continue from the last exercise. (Fig-21)

Continue exhaling and squat down. (Fig-22) The hands move down as if they are scooping water up.

Inhale and stand up as you raise the arms up the front and over the head. Look up at the hands. (Fig-23)

Exhale and separate the hands and move them down to the sides, imagining the water that you scooped trickling down your body relaxing you. As the hands move down the head also moves down to look straight ahead. (Fig-21)

Repeat this 3 times. Then move into the next exercise.

This exercise is also called Crane Washing Itself.

If you can not come to a full squat don't force it. Just go as low as is comfortable.

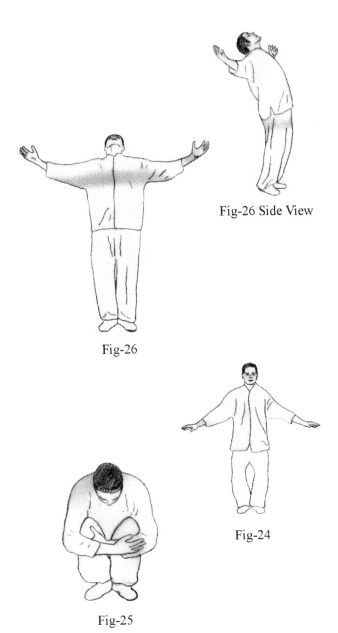

Fig-26 Side View

Fig-26

Fig-24

Fig-25

B. Squatting Crane II

Continuing the exhale from the last exercise (Fig-24), squat down and hug your knees. (Fig-25)

Inhale stand up and extend the arms out to the side at shoulder level and bend the body back slightly so that the chest and the palms face towards the sky. (Fig-26) Pause for a moment. Note- during this small pause you are holding your breath.

Exhale squat down a second time and hug the knees. (Fig-25)
Inhale and lean back a little bit further this time. (Fig-26) Pause for a moment. Note- during this small pause you are holding your breath.

Exhale and squat a third time and hug the knees. (Fig-25) Inhale stand up and lean back a little further than you did last time. (Fig-26) As you hold this position use the hips by rotating them left and right to rotate the chest and move the arms up and down several times. Note- the chest and arms remain stationary. The movement is all from the hips turning. During this rotating movement you are holding your breath.

Then exhale and return to the Crane Stance with the hands on the lower abdomen.

If you can not come to a full squat don't force it. Just go as low as is comfortable. Do not strain the breath or become out of breath. Hold the breath for only as long is as comfortable.

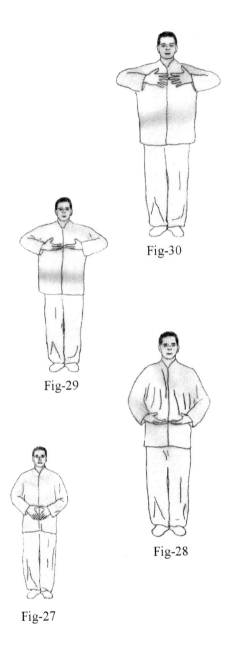

Fig-30

Fig-29

Fig-28

Fig-27

58

5. Breathing Crane II

From the Crane Stance (Fig-27) bring your palms face up in front of the lower abdomen with the middle fingers touching. (Fig-28) Inhale as you raise the palms to chest level. (Fig-29) Hold the breath as you turn the palms to face the chest and make small circles over the heart area. (Fig-30) The circles move up your right side and down your left side.

Turn the palms so that they are face up in front of the chest. (Fig-29) Exhale as you lower the hands so that they are in front of the lower abdomen. (Fig-28)

Inhale and raise the hands to chest level. (Fig-29) Turn the palms so that they face the chest. (Fig-30) Hold the breath. This time make slightly larger circles over the heart region. The circles move up your right side and down your left side. Turn the palms so that they are face up in front of the chest. (Fig-29) Exhale the palms back down to the level of the lower abdomen. (Fig-28)

Inhale and raise the hands to chest level. (Fig-29) Turn the palms so that they face the chest. (Fig-30) Hold the breath. This time circle the entire chest region. The circles move up your right side and down your left side. Turn the palms so that they are face up in front of the chest. (Fig-29) Exhale the palms back down to the level of the lower abdomen. (Fig-28) Return to the Crane Stance with the palms on the lower abdomen. (Fig-27)

Hold the breath and circle the arms only as long as is comfortable. There is not a set number of times to circle the hands. While circling the hands, the middle fingers stay in contact and the forearms stay in a straight line. The body does not move while the arms are circling.

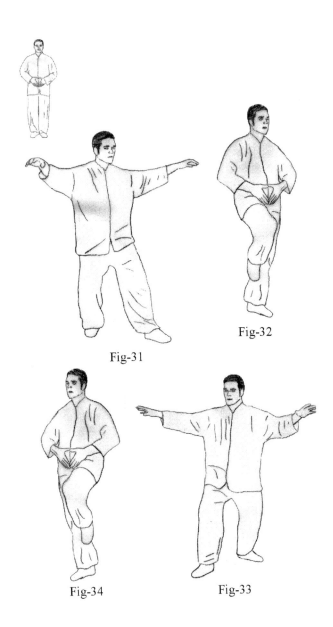

Fig-31

Fig-32

Fig-34

Fig-33

60

6. Stepping Crane

A. Stepping Crane I

From the Crane Stance, take a step with your left foot as you inhale and separate your hands and move them up to the side so that they are at shoulder level. The palms should be facing downward. (Fig-31)

Exhale as you bring your hands back to your lower abdomen like in the Crane Stance and you raise your right leg so that the right foot is next to the left knee. (Fig-32)

Inhale and take a step with the right foot as you separate your hands and move them up to the side so that they are at shoulder level. The palms should be facing downward. (Fig-33)

Exhale as you bring your hands back to your lower abdomen like in the Crane Stance and raise your left leg so that the left foot is next to the right knee. (Fig-34)

Repeat as many times as you wish.

To finish, as you exhale, return to the Crane Stance rather than standing on one leg.

Each time you are standing on one leg pause for a moment. You should feel steady. Over time your balance will improve. Think of a Crane standing on one leg. The Crane is poised and elegant. This is your goal.

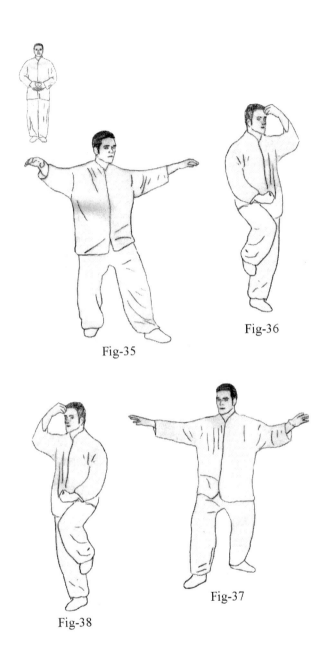

Fig-35

Fig-36

Fig-37

Fig-38

B. Stepping Crane II

This is the same as the first walking exercise only the position of the hands is different when you are standing on one leg.

From the Crane Stance, take a step with your left foot as you inhale and separate your hands and move them up to the side so that they are at shoulder level with the palms facing downward. (Fig-35) Exhale as you raise your right leg so that the right foot is next to the left knee. The hands form Crane's Beaks. The right hand moves so the fingers point towards the lower abdomen. The left hand moves so the fingers point towards the forehead. (Fig-36)

Inhale and take a step with the right foot as and separate your hands and move them up to the side so that they are at shoulder level with the palms facing downward. (Fig-37) Exhale as you raise your left leg so that the left foot is next to the right knee. The hands form Crane's Beaks. The left hand moves so the fingers point towards the lower abdomen. The right hand moves so the fingers point towards the forehead. (Fig-38)

Repeat as many times as you wish. You may also practice with the hands reversed.

To finish, step and raise the arms as you inhale. Exhale, return to the crane stance instead of standing on one leg.

Each time you are standing on one leg pause for a moment. You should feel steady. Again your goal is to be as poised and elegant as a Crane standing on one leg.

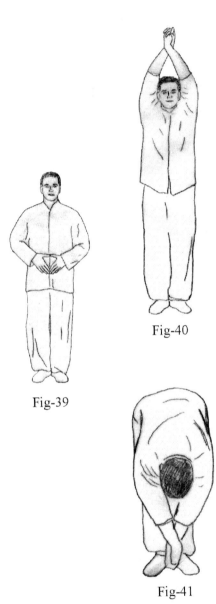

Fig-39

Fig-40

Fig-41

64

7. Beak in the Mud

Start from the Crane Stance. (Fig-39)

Raise the arms up the sides so that they meet over the head. Interlace the fingers of the palms with the right palm facing the right side and the left palm facing the left side. (Fig-40)

Bend your knees slightly. Then bend your body forward at the waist. Straighten your knees and let your body hang from the waist. (Fig-41)

The top of the head should be facing the ground. From this position, try to relax your spine completely. It should feel as if the spine is hanging from the hips. Hanging the spine in this way allows the vertebrae to relax and lengthen. This position is counter to the normal force of gravity that is placed on our vertebrae while we are standing upright.

You might also feel a gentle stretch on the back of the legs.

Breathe naturally. From here, go directly into the next exercise.

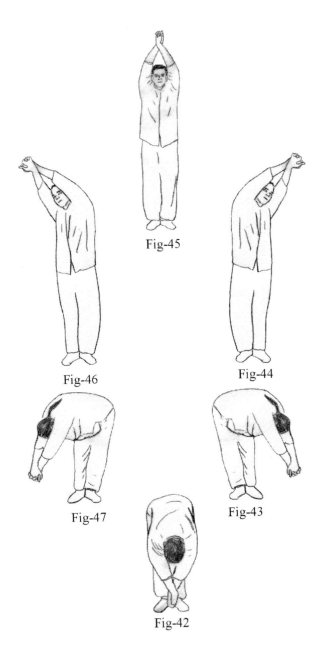

Fig-45

Fig-46

Fig-44

Fig-47

Fig-43

Fig-42

66

8. Circle Crane

Start from the Beak in the Mud posture. (Fig-42) Bend the knees slightly. Then inhale and circle your body up the left side. (Fig-43 and Fig-44) As you finish the inhale your body should be straight, knees still bent slightly, and the hands still interlaced over the head. (Fig-45) Then exhale as you circle down the right side. (Fig-46 and Fig-47) Then straighten the legs as you hang and rest in the Beak in the Mud posture. (Fig-42)

Then bend the knees slightly, inhale and circle your body up the right side. (Fig-47 and Fig-46) As you finish the inhale your body should be straight, knees still bent slightly, and the hands still interlaced over the head. (Fig45) Then exhale and circle down the left side. (Fig-44 and Fig-43) Then straighten the legs as you hang and rest in the Beak in the Mud posture. (Fig-42)

Start with 1 circle on each side and work your way up to 3 circles on each side. Alternate from side to side and rest in the Beak in the Mud posture in between circles.

To end, bend the knees and inhale as you bring the body up to the front by rolling your spine up vertebrae by vertebrae starting with your sacrum. When you finish the inhale your body should be straight, knees still bend slightly, and the hands still interlaced over the head. (Fig-45) Then exhale, unlock your fingers and lower the hands down the sides to return to the Crane Stance.

It is important to bend the knees before circling the body or bringing the body back up. This takes the stress off your lower back during these movements.

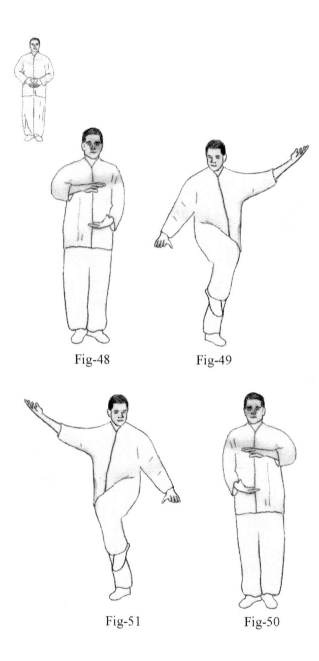

Fig-48   Fig-49

Fig-51   Fig-50

68

9. Basic Crane

From the Crane Stance, move your hands in front of you as if you were holding a ball. The right hand is on top and the left hand is on the bottom. (Fig-48)

Then inhale, turn the body so it faces the left front corner. Separate the hands, left hand at head level palm up and right palm face down at hip level. Raise the right foot so it is by the left knee. Look at the right hand. (Fig-49)

Exhale, drop the right foot and bring the hands to the front like you are holding a ball with the left hand on top and the right hand on the bottom. The feet are in the same position they were when you started the exercise in the Crane Stance. (Fig-50)

Then inhale, turn the body so it faces the right front corner. Separate the hands, right hand at head level palm up and left palm face down at hip level. Raise the left foot so it is by the right knee. Look at the left hand. (Fig-51)

Exhale, drop the right foot and bring the hands to the front like you are holding a ball with the right hand on top and the left hand on the bottom. (Fig-48)

Repeat this 3 to 5 times. Then continue into the last exercise.

Remember to coordinate the speed of the movement with the breathing. As you move the arms you should feel the resistance of the air as if your arms are the wings of a Crane.

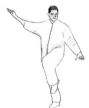

Fig-52

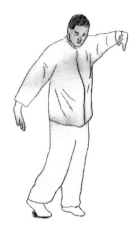

Fig-53

Fig-54

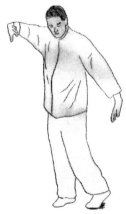

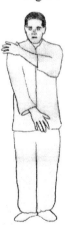

Fig-56

Fig-55

70

10. White Crane Spreads Wings

Start from the last posture of Basic Crane. (Fig-52) Exhale and drop the left foot. Move the left hand to the body's centerline with the palm facing the body. Move the right hand across so that the palm faces the left shoulder. (Fig-53)

Inhale and wipe the right hand down the left arm (the palm does not touch the arm but is very close). Turn the body to the left front and raise the left arm with the palm facing away from the body. Lift the right heel and turn the right foot so that the heel is facing to the right side. The right palm faces the right side with the fingers pointed towards the floor. Look at the right hand. (Fig-54)

Exhale and move the right foot back into a Crane Stance. Move the right hand to the body's centerline with the palm facing the body. Move the left hand across so that the palm faces the right shoulder. (Fig-55)

Inhale, wipe the left hand down the right arm (the palm does not touch the arm but is very close). Turn the body to the right front and raise the right arm with the palm facing away from the body. Lift the left heel and turn the left foot so that the heel is facing to the left side. The left palm faces the left side with the fingers pointed towards the floor. Look at the left hand. (Fig-56)

Repeat this movement 3 to 5 times. On the last one exhale and return to the Crane Stance.

This movement is also called Crane Washing Its' Wing. Make sure to coordinate the breathing with the movements and feel the resistance of the air as you move your arms.

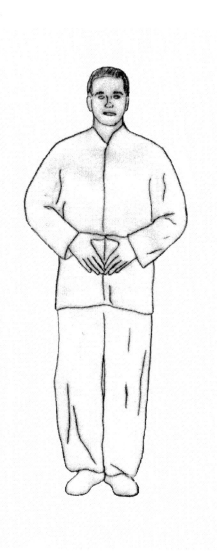

Finishing The Crane Frolics Qi Gong

When you finish the last exercises you are back in the Crane Stance.

Stand and concentrate on your breathing for a while. (Fig-57)

Then you can end your practice by gently walking around the room. As you walk you can keep your hands at the lower abdomen. Then gently relax your arms to your sides as you walk for a bit more.

Then end your practice.

Bear Frolics
Qi Gong

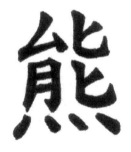

Introduction

The Bear Frolics Qi Gong Exercises are practiced from a grounded stance and consists of turning motions that imitate the movements of a Bear.

The Bear exercises belong to the Water element and strengthen the Kidneys and Urogenital system.

Like the Crane exercises, the movements of this set should be coordinated with the breathing. Never strain or become out of breath. The key is to be relaxed and natural at all times.

The Bear Stance can be very strenuous, especially when you hold it at a lower level. When performing this set try to stay at the same level. You want to avoid having to raise your body in the middle of the set because your legs are tired. In the beginning take a higher stance and as you progress you will be able to take a lower stance.

Hand Positions

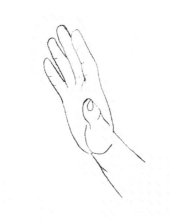

Palm

The fingers are naturally extended and the center of the palm should be slightly hollow. (Fig-58)

The hand should not be too straight or stiff or too curved or bent.

Extending the fingers in this way lets the Qi and the blood flow to the extremities of the body.

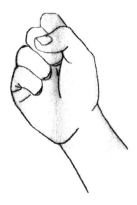

Loose Fist

Make a fist but do not clench the hand. (Fig-59)

Use only enough force to keep the fist closed.

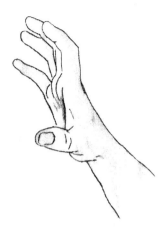

Bear Claw

Start with the fingers extended.

Then, slightly curve the fingers and thumb as if you were about to take hold of something. (Fig-60)

Do not bend the fingers too much.

There should be some tension in the hand but you should not have to strain to hold the position. Also the hand is not held stiffly.

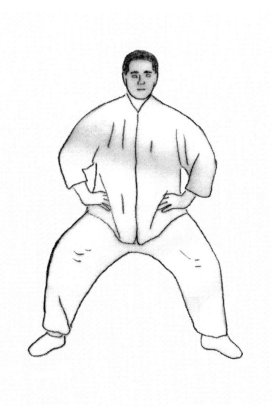

Bear Stance

Stand with the feet slightly wider than shoulder width apart to about double shoulder width apart. The feet should be pointed out slightly so that the angle between to two feet is between 60 and 90 degrees.

Bend the knees and relax the pelvis so that it naturally drops forward slightly, straightening the lower back. (Fig-61)

Curl the tongue upwards so that the tip touches the upper palette.

Note: The knees should always be in line with the toes throughout these exercises.

The width of the stance and the depth the knees are bent depends on the practitioner. The wider your stance is and the deeper you bend your knees, the harder the physical workout.

Do not bend your knees so deep that your hips are below your knees. The deepest position should be with the thighs parallel to the ground and the hips and knees at the same height.

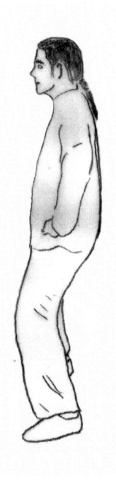

As you stand in this position try to feel that your spine is elongated by both stretching up and down.

This stretching feeling is very subtle and should not be forced.

By relaxing your hips and letting your pelvis drop naturally forward you are lengthening the lower part of your spine. When the pelvis drops naturally forward the hips should be tucked slightly as if you were about to sit. Again there should be no tension in the hips.

To stretch the upper parts of the spine try to imagine that you are suspended from above. Let the entire body relax and "hang" as if by a string. Make sure that there is no tension in the neck. The proper position for the neck is with the chin pushed back and slightly down as if you are trying to touch the back of the neck to your shirt collar.

It is important to remember to always keep your knees in line with the toes and to always keep the back straight.

Another important point in the Bear frolics Qi Gong is the difference between the hips and the waist. If we refer to the hips we are talking about the actual hip bones or the place where the legs and pelvis meet. The waist is the portion above the hips and below the ribs.

If the instructions say to turn the waist then the hips should stay stationary. Turn your waist only as far as is comfortable. Turning in is manner stimulates the organs in the abdomen and helps to strengthen the waist and Kidneys.

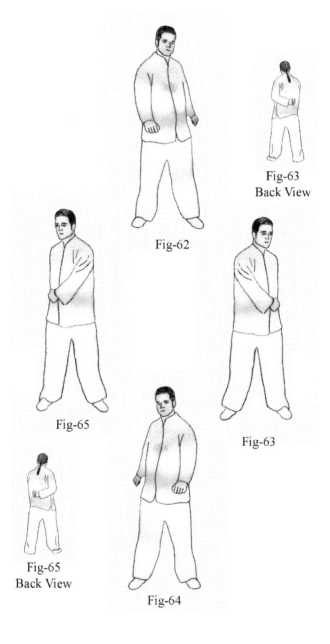

Fig-63
Back View

Fig-62

Fig-65

Fig-63

Fig-65
Back View

Fig-64

86

1. Flopping Bear

Stand in a higher Bear Stance with the feet about shoulder width apart. Make your hands into loose fists and keep your arms relaxed by your side.

Turn your body to the left. (Fig-62) The turning should be done with enough speed so that your relaxed arms will swing with the movement. The left arm will swing behind the body and the left fist will tap the lower back. The right arm will also swing to the left but the fist will tap the lower abdomen. (Fig-63)

Then turn the body to the right and let the relaxed arms swing to the right. (Fig-64) The right arm will swing behind the body and the fist will tap the lower back. The left arm will swing to the right and the left fist will tap the lower abdomen. (Fig-65)

Keep the arms relaxed and the fists loose. The movement of the arms should be generated from the waist and the hips turning. Do not tap yourself too hard. This exercise should feel comfortable. As you turn the body back and forth, keep the weight centered between the feet. Keep your feet on the ground and your knees in line with your toes.

Swing the body for a couple minutes.

This exercise can be practiced separately and is a good warm up for any physical activity.

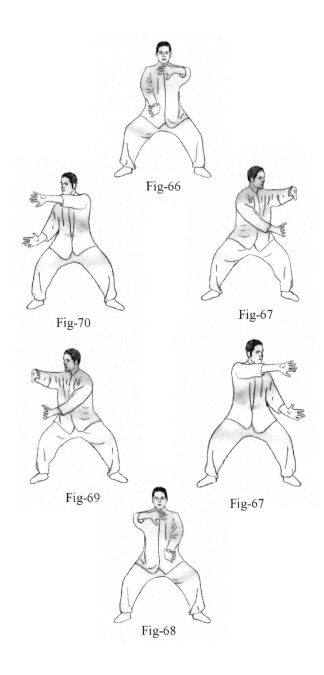

Fig-66

Fig-70

Fig-67

Fig-69

Fig-67

Fig-68

2. Fishing Bear

A. Fishing Bear I

Stand in the Bear Stance. Hands are in Bear Claws. Extend the left hand out in front of you at chest level and turn the palm so that it faces outward. The fingers should point to the right. Extend the left hand out in front of you at the level of your lower abdomen. The palm should face outward and the fingers should point to the right. (Fig-66)

Inhale and use your waist to turn the upper body towards the left. The hands follow the movement of the body. (Fig-67)

Drop the left hand to the level of the lower abdomen and bring the right hand up to the level of the chest. Turn the hands so that the palms face outward and the fingers of both hands should point to the left. (Fig-68)

Use your waist to turn your body towards the right. The hands follow the movement of the upper body. Exhale to the center (Fig-68) and Inhale as you turn to the right (Fig69)

Drop the right hand to the level of the lower abdomen and bring the left hand up to the level of the chest. Turn the hands so that the palms face outward and the fingers of both hands should point to the right. (Fig-70)

Repeat this movement 3 to 5 times.

You should imagine that you are dragging your fingers through water like a Bear fishing. As your turn left and right, remember to keep the weight centered between the legs and the hips and knees stationary.

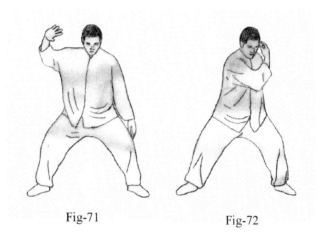

Fig-71   Fig-72

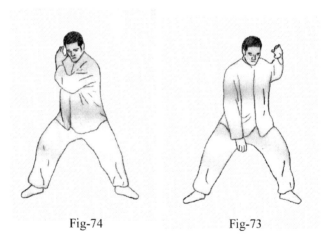

Fig-74   Fig-73

90

B. Fishing Bear II

Start in the Bear Stance. The arms are relaxed and hanging to your sides. Bring the right arm up next to the right ear. (Fig-71)

Keep the arm relaxed and let it swing down in an arc and up over the left shoulder. Imagine you are a Bear swatting a fish out of a river. The body should move slightly with this movement. (Fig-72)

Move the left hand up to the left ear and let the right arm go back to the right side. (Fig-73)

Let the left hand swing down in an arc and up over the right shoulder. The body should move slightly with this movement. (Fig-74)

Breathe naturally.

Repeat this movement 3 to 5 times.

It is important to keep the body and arms relaxed throughout this movement.

Let the arms swing and keep the weight centered between the feet.

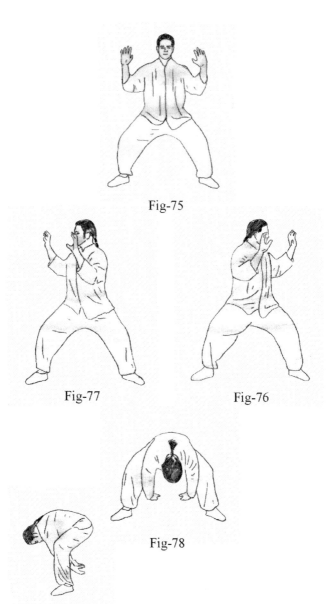

Fig-75

Fig-77

Fig-76

Fig-78

Fig-78 Side View

3. Turning and Tipping Bear

Stand in the Bear Stance. Bring your Bear Claws up to the front and slightly wider than shoulder width. The hands should be slightly higher than the shoulders. The palms should face the front and the elbows should be dropped downward and relaxed. Make sure there is no tension in the shoulders. The hands and arms should be held slightly in front of the body. (Fig-75)

Inhale and use the waist to turn the upper body to the left. The hands remain still in relation to the body. (Fig-76)

Exhale and turn back to the front. (Fig-75)

Inhale and use the waist to turn to the right. The hands remain still in relation to the body. (Fig-77)

Exhale and turn back to the front. (Fig-75)

Repeat this 3 times.

Then, keeping the knees bent, exhale and bend the body forward at the waist. Use your hands to reach through your legs and behind yourself. (Fig-78)

Inhale back up to the beginning posture. (Fig-75)

In the beginning repeat this whole sequence 1 time and gradually work up to 3 repetitions.

Turn your body only as far as is comfortable. The hips and the knees should not move during the turn.

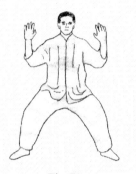

Fig-79

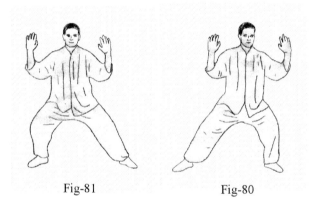

Fig-81   Fig-80

94

4. Squatting Bear

Continue from the last exercise. Your Bear Claws held up to the front and slightly wider than shoulder width. The hands should be slightly higher than the shoulders. The palms should face the front and the elbows should be dropped downward and relaxed. Make sure there is no tension in the shoulders.(Fig-79)

Slowly shift the weight over to the left leg. (Fig-80)

Then slowly shift the weight back to the center. (Fig-79)

Then slowly shift the weight over to the right leg. (Fig-81)

Then slowly shift the weight back to the center. (Fig-79)

Repeat this 3 to 5 times.

The body should not move up and down when the weight is shifted. The movement should be a slow even horizontal movement of the body, the slower the better. The breathing should be natural.

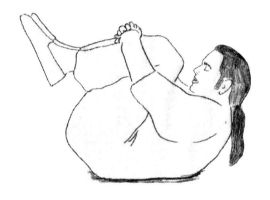

96

5. Rolling Bear

Lie on your back.

Bring your knees up to your chest.

Hold your knees with your arms/hands.

Raise the head towards the knees rounding the back.

Gently rock back and forth and side to side for about a minute. (Fig-82)

Breathe naturally.

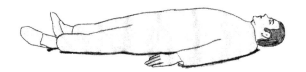

6. *Hibernating Bear*

Lie on your back.

The feet should be separated to about shoulder width. The hands should be relaxed with the palms facing the ground. (Fig-83)

Close your eyes and feel your body relax into the earth. Your body should be fully supported by the ground. You should not be using any tension to hold yourself up.

Scan your body for tension. Start with your head and work down your body to the feet. Relax any tension away. Scan your body 3 times from the head to the feet, relaxing away any tension.

After you have relaxed away all your tension stay in this position and concentrate on your breathing. One method is to practice the Crane Breathing that was descried earlier. As you inhale feel you abdomen expand. Exhale and the abdomen will relax back to its original position. Try to make the breathing slow and relaxed. But do not force it.

Concentrate on your breathing for several minutes.

This exercise may be practiced by itself. When this posture is practiced by itself you can relax and concentrate on your breathing for as long as you like.

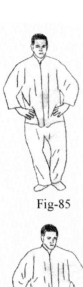

Fig-85

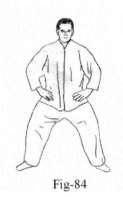

Fig-84

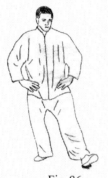

Fig-86

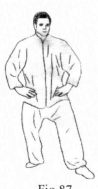

Fig-87

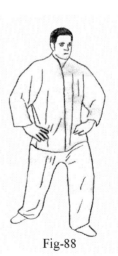

Fig-88

7. *Bear Crosses the Ice*

A. Bear Crosses the Ice I

Start in the Bear Stance with the hands at the hips, finger pointing forward. (Fig-84)

Shift the weight to the right leg. Bring the left foot close to the right foot. (Fig-85)

Then step out with the left foot. The heel touches the ground first but has no weight on it. (Fig-86)

After the heel touches the ground, drop the toes down but still with no weight on the foot. (Fig-87)

After the foot is flat on the ground with no weight on it, slowly shift the weight onto the left leg. (Fig-88)

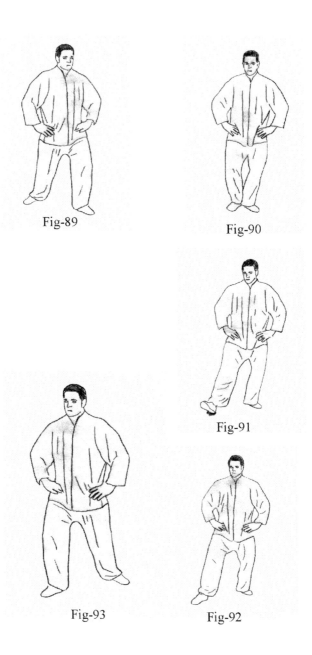

Fig-89

Fig-90

Fig-91

Fig-93

Fig-92

To take another step, bring the right foot up to the left foot.(Fig-90)

Then step out with the right foot. The heel touches the ground first but has no weight on it. (Fig-91)

After the heel touches the ground, drop the toes down but still with no weight on the foot. (Fig-92)

After the foot is flat on the ground with no weight on it, slowly shift the weight onto the right leg. (Fig-93)

Repeat as many times as you wish.

Breathe naturally and make these movements slow and even. Feel the weight sink all the way down to the ground and stay at the same level as you walk. Try not to bob up and down.

Have complete control over your steps and shift the weight slowly as if you were walking on ice, but at the same time you should feel very heavy like a bear.

To end this exercise, instead of stepping out, step back into the Bear Stance.

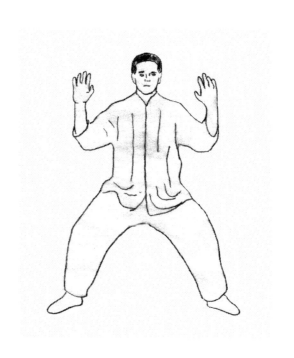

B. Bear Crosses the Ice II

Stand in the Bear Stance. Bring your Bear Claws up to the front and slightly wider than shoulder width. The hands should be slightly higher than the shoulders. The palms should face the front and the elbows should be dropped downward and relaxed. Make sure there is no tension in the shoulders. The hands and arms should be held slightly in front of the body.(Fig-94)

The steps are the same as before but now the upper body is held in this position.

You will notice that with the hands held in this position it adds a slightly new dimension to the walking exercise. In the beginning it will be harder to relax and sink all the body weight down through the feet and into the earth.

Breathe naturally and make these movements slow and even. Stay at the same level as you walk. Try not to bob up and down.

Have complete control over your steps and shift the weight slowly as if you were walking on ice, but at the same time you should feel very heavy like a bear.

To end this exercise, instead of stepping out, step back into the Bear Stance.

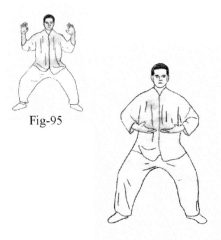

Fig-95

Fig-96

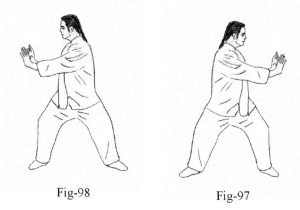

Fig-98   Fig-97

106

8. Pushing Bear

A. Bear Pushes to the Side

Continue from the last exercises. (Fig-95)
Bring your hands down so they are palm up between the solar plexus and the navel. The fingers should be pointing at each other. (Fig-96)

Inhale. Use your waist to turn your body to the left and push the palms out at chest level. (Fig-97)

Exhale and return to the original position. (Fig-96)

Inhale. Use your waist to turn the body to the right and push the palms out at chest level. (Fig-98)

Exhale and return to the original position. (Fig-96)

Turn your body only as far as is comfortable. The hips and the knees should not move during the turn. Coordinate the movement with the breathing.

Then move on to the next part of the exercise.

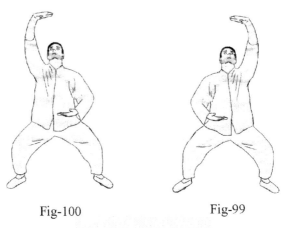

Fig-100   Fig-99

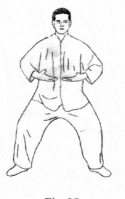

Fig-98

B. Bear Pushes Up

Continue from the last exercise with the palms facing upward in front of the body. (Fig-98)

Inhale and raise the left hand up and over the head. As the hand is coming up turn it over so that the palm pushes upward. Tilt your head slightly so that you can look at your hand. Make sure you do not come up in your stance while pushing the hand up. (Fig-99)

Exhale and drop the left palm back into the original position. As the hand returns to in front of the body, the head should be looking straight ahead. (Fig-98)

Inhale and raise the right hand up and over the head. As the hand is coming up turn it over so that the palm pushes upward. Tilt your head slightly so that you can look at your hand. Make sure you do not come up in your stance while pushing the hand up. (Fig-100)

Exhale and drop the left palm back into the original position. As the hand returns to in front of the body, the head should be looking straight ahead. (Fig-98)

Then move into the next exercise.

Remember to coordinate the movement with the breathing.

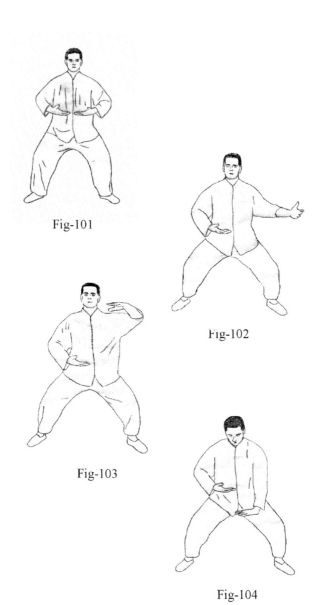

Fig-101

Fig-102

Fig-103

Fig-104

110

C. Bear Pushes Down

Continue from the last exercise. (Fig-101)

Inhale and circle the left hand out to the side, up and around to shoulder level. Your hand should move in a circular motion. Your hand should end at shoulder level with the palm facing down and the fingers pointing to the right. (Fig-102 and Fig-103)

Exhale and push the palm down in front of you. Look at your hand. (Fig-104)

Remember to coordinate the movement with the breath. Do not change the height of your stance through the movement.

Continue to the next part of this exercise.

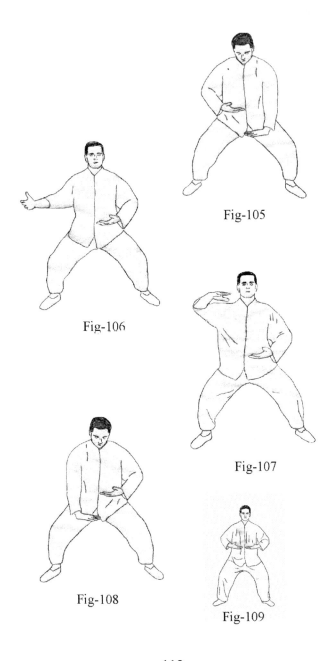

Fig-105

Fig-106

Fig-107

Fig-108

Fig-109

112

C. Bear Pushes Down (continued)

Continue from the last exercise. (Fig-105)

Inhale and circle the right hand out to the side, up and around to shoulder level. Your hand should move in a circular motion. Your hand should end at shoulder level with the palm facing down and the fingers pointing to the left. At the same time move your left hand up so that it is palm up in front of the body. (Fig-106 and Fig-107)

Exhale and push the palm down in front of you. Look at your hand. (Fig-108)

Then inhale and bring the right hand back up in front of the body with the palm facing upward. (Fig-109)

Remember to coordinate the movement with the breath. Do not change the height of your stance through the movement.

You have just completed one set (Bear Pushes to the Side, Up, and Down).

Do 3-5 sets of this exercise.

Then move into the next exercise.

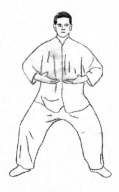

Fig-110

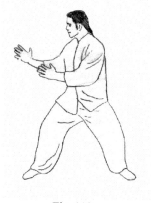

Fig-112

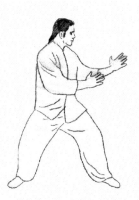

Fig-111

114

9. Marauding Bear

A. Bear Roll Back

Continue from the last exercise with the palms in front of the lower abdomen and the fingers pointing at each other. (Fig-110)

Inhale and use the waist to turn your body to the left. Shift the weight so that the right leg has slightly more weight than the left leg. As you shift the weight the hips should turn slightly as well. Extend the hands to the left with the fingertips pointing away from the body and the palms facing each other. The left hand should be extended slightly more than the right hand. (Fig-111)

Exhale and return to the original position. (Fig-110)

Inhale and use the waist to turn your body to the right. Shift the weight so that the left leg has slightly more weight than the right leg. As you shift the weight the hips should turn slightly as well. Extend the hands to the right with the fingertips pointing away from the body and the palms facing each other. The right hand should be extended slightly more than the left hand. (Fig-112)

Exhale and return to the original position. (Fig-110)

Repeat this movement 3 times. Then move into the next part of the exercise.

Coordinate the movement with the breathing.

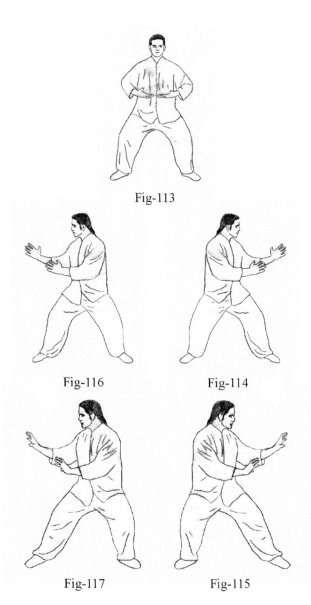

Fig-113

Fig-116　　　　　Fig-114

Fig-117　　　　　Fig-115

B. Mauling Bear

Continue from the last exercise with the palms in front of the lower abdomen and the fingers pointing at each other. (Fig-113) Inhale and use the waist to turn your body to the left. Shift the weight so that the right leg has slightly more weight than the left leg. As you shift the weight the hips should turn slightly as well. Extend the hands to the left with the fingertips pointing away from the body and the palms facing each other. The left hand should be extended slightly more than the right hand. (Fig-114)

Then shift a little more weight onto the right leg and turn the palms so that they face away from the body and form relaxed Bear Claws by separating and bending the fingers. (Fig-115) During this movement there is no breathing. Exhale and return to the original position. (Fig-113)

Inhale and use the waist to turn your body to the right. Shift the weight so that the left leg has slightly more weight than the right leg. As you shift the weight the hips should turn slightly as well. Extend the hands to the right with the fingertips pointing away from the body and the palms facing each other. The right hand should be extended slightly more than the left hand. (Fig-116)

Then shift a little more weight onto the left leg and turn the palms so that they face away from the body and form relaxed Bear Claws by separating and bending the fingers. (Fig-117) During this movement there is no breathing. Exhale and return to the original position. (Fig-113)

Repeat this movement 3 times. Then move into the next part of the exercise.

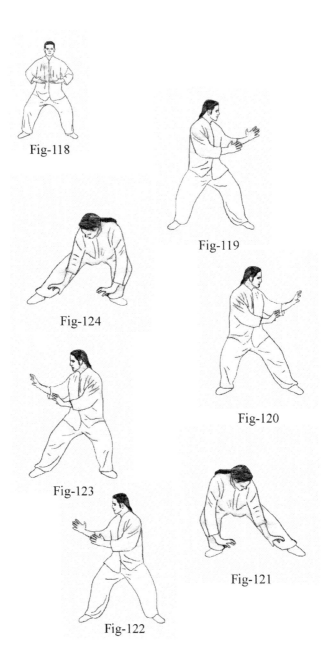

Fig-118

Fig-119

Fig-124

Fig-120

Fig-123

Fig-121

Fig-122

118

C. Bear Take Down

Continue from the last exercise. (Fig-118) The first two movements are the same as before. Turn to the left and extend the hands as you inhale. (Fig-119) Then turn the hands into Bear Claws as you shift the weight a little more. (Fig-120)

Then, exhale and shift almost all the weight to the right leg. Bend the body slightly forward and pull your hands down and back close to the floor. (Fig-121)

Inhale and use the waist to turn your body to the right. Shift the weight so that the left leg has slightly more weight than the right leg. Extend the hands to the right with the fingertips pointing away from the body and the palms facing each other. The right hand should be extended slightly more than the left hand. (Fig-122)

Repeat these movements on this side. (Fig-123 and Fig124)

Repeat this exercise 3 times.

On the last repetition you will inhale and come up to the left with the hands extended. (Fig-119)

To end, exhale and bring the hands back in front of the lower abdomen with the palms facing up. (Fig-118)

Then move into the last exercise.

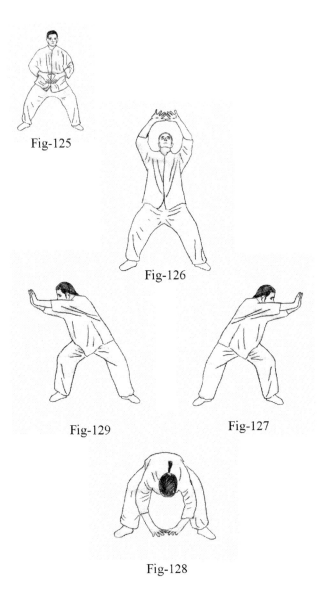

Fig-125

Fig-126

Fig-129

Fig-127

Fig-128

120

10. Looking Bear

Continue from the last exercise, place your hands on your stomach. The thumbs and the index fingers are touching so that the hands form a triangle with the thumbs at the bellybutton and the fingers pointing down. (Fig-125)

Bring the hands away from the body and up over the head. The thumbs and index fingers should still be touching. Look through the triangle that is formed by this hand position. As you move the hands up over the head move them in a zigzag or "S" pattern. Follow this movement with your vision. Let the body follow the vision. (Fig-126)

Exhale and circle the body down the left.
(Fig-127 and Fig-128)
Inhale and circle the body up the right side.
(Fig-129 and Fig-126)
Circle the body 3 times. The vision should be directed through the triangle formed by the hands. The lower body stays stationary through this movement.

Then exhale and circle the body down to the right.
(Fig-129 and Fig-128)
Inhale and circle the body up to the light.
(Fig-127 and Fig-126)
Circle the body in this direction 3 times.

To end, move the hands from above the head (Fig-126) to the lower abdomen. (Fig-125)

The range of motion on this exercise should be comfortable. Do not over do it.

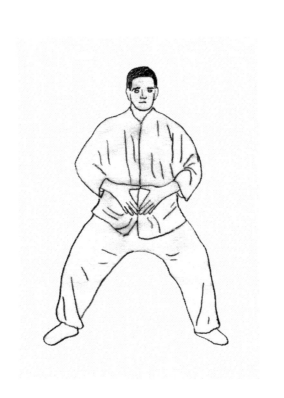

Finishing The Bear Frolics Qi Gong

When you finish the last exercises you are back in the Bear Stance and the hands are on the lower abdomen. The index finger and thumb should be touching. The thumbs meet at the navel and the fingers are pointing downward.

Stand and concentrate on your breathing for a while. (Fig-130)

Then you can end your practice by gently walking around the room. As you walk you can keep your hands at the lower abdomen. Then gently relax your arms to your sides as you walk for a bit more.

Then end your practice.

Crane Frolics Qi Gong Exercise List

1. Windmill Crane
2. Breathing Crane
3. Soaring Crane
       A. Soaring Crane I
       B. Soaring Crane II
       C. Soaring Crane III
4. Squatting Crane
       A. Squatting Crane I
       B. Squatting Crane II
5. Breathing Crane II
6. Stepping Crane
       A. Stepping Crane I
       B. Stepping Crane II
7. Beak in the Mud
8. Circle Crane
9. Basic Crane
10. White Crane Spreads Wings

Bear Frolics Qi Gong Exercise List

1. Flopping Bear
2. Fishing Bear
   - A. Fishing Bear I
   - B. Fishing Bear II
3. Turning and Tipping Bear
4. Squatting Bear
5. Rolling Bear
6. Hibernating Bear
7. Bear Crosses the Ice
   - A. Bear Crosses the Ice I
   - B. Bear Crosses the Ice II
8. Pushing Bear
   - A. Bear Pushes to the Side
   - B. Bear Pushes Up
   - C. Bear Pushes Down
9. Marauding Bear
   - A. Bear Roll Back
   - B. Mauling Bear
   - C. Bear Take Down
10. Looking Bear

About the Author

Franklin Fick has been teaching Kung Fu and Qi Gong since 1993. He teaches Yang style Taiji Quan, Xing Yi Quan, Ba Gua Zhang, Shaolin Kung Fu, Qi Gong, Meditation, and Tui-Na.

Franklin also has a Master Degree in Traditional Chinese Medicine.

For information about classes or seminars please visit:
www.spiritdragoninstitute.com

For information about other great products including books and future please visit:
www.shenlongpub.com

8682850R0

Made in the USA
Lexington, KY
23 February 2011